AKALINE DIET

Evidence Based-Review

Joan kim

Table of Contents

CHAPTER 1

The alkaline diet may aid health by restricting processed meals and selling extra whole meals. However it does now not help fight disease through affecting your body's pH tiers.

What is the alkaline diet?

The alkaline food regimen is also known as the acid-alkaline weight loss plan or alkaline ash food plan.

Its premise is that your food regimen can adjust the pH price —

the dimension of acidity or alkalinity — of your frame.

Your metabolism — the conversion of food into electricity — is once in a while compared to fireplace. Each contain a chemical reaction that breaks down a strong mass.

But, the chemical reactions in your body take place in a gradual and controlled manner.

Whilst matters burn, an ash residue is left behind. In addition, the foods you eat depart an "ash" residue referred to as metabolic waste.

This metabolic waste may be alkaline, neutral, or acidic. Proponents of this weight loss plan claim that metabolic waste can without delay affect your body's acidity.

In other words, in case you eat foods that leave acidic ash, it makes your blood extra acidic. In case you consume meals that go away alkaline ash, it makes your blood more alkaline.

In step with the acid-ash speculation, acidic ash is notion to make you prone to contamination and disease, while alkaline ash is taken into consideration protective.

With the aid of deciding on more alkaline foods, you ought to be capable of "alkalize" your frame and enhance your fitness.

Food additives that go away an acidic ash include protein, phosphate, and sulfur, even as alkaline additives encompass calcium, magnesium, and potassium.

Positive food corporations are considered acidic, alkaline, or neutral:

Acidic: meat, poultry, fish, dairy, eggs, grains, alcohol

Neutral: natural fats, starches, and sugars

Alkaline: end result, nuts, legumes, and vegetables

Summary

In step with proponents of the alkaline food regimen, the metabolic waste — or ash — left from the burning of meals can directly have an effect on the acidity or alkalinity of your frame.

Normal pH degrees for your body

When discussing the alkaline weight loss plan, it's essential to recognize pH.

Positioned simply, pH is a dimension of the way acidic or alkaline some thing is.

The pH price stages from zero–14:

Acidic: zero.0–6.9

Impartial: 7.Zero

Alkaline (or fundamental): 7.1–14.0

Many proponents of this diet advocate that humans screen the pH in their urine to ensure that it's miles alkaline (over 7) and not acidic (underneath 7).

However, it's important to note that pH varies substantially within your body. At the same time as some elements are acidic, others are alkaline — there's no set stage.

Your belly is loaded with hydrochloric acid, giving it a pH of two–three. Five, that's enormously acidic. This acidity is necessary to break down meals.

However, human blood is usually slightly alkaline, with a pH of 7.36–7.Forty four.

While your blood pH falls out of the ordinary range, it is able to be fatal if left untreated.

However, this only takes place at some point of sure sickness states, which includes ketoacidosis caused by diabetes, hunger, or alcohol consumption.

The pH cost measures a substance's acidity or alkalinity. For example, stomach acid is quite acidic, whilst blood is barely alkaline.

Meals influences the pH of your urine, however not your blood

It's vital in your health that the pH of your blood remains consistent.

If it have been to fall outside of the everyday variety, your cells would forestall operating and you will die very quickly if untreated.

For that reason, your frame has many powerful approaches to closely regulate its pH stability. This is referred to as acid-base homeostasis.

In fact, it's nearly impossible for food to change the pH fee of blood in healthy human beings, even though tiny fluctuations can occur inside the normal range.

But, food can change the pH fee of your urine — even though the effect is relatively variable.

Excreting acids to your urine is one of the fundamental ways your frame regulates its blood pH.

In case you eat a massive steak, your urine may be greater acidic numerous hours later as your body eliminates the metabolic waste out of your system.

Therefore, urine pH is a poor indicator of average body pH and standard fitness. It may additionally be inspired by means of elements aside from your diet.

Summary

Your body tightly regulates blood pH stages. In healthful people, weight loss program doesn't significantly have an effect on blood pH, but it may trade urine pH.

Acid-forming ingredients and osteoporosis

Osteoporosis is a innovative bone ailment characterised through a decrease in bone mineral content.

It's mainly common amongst postmenopausal women and might substantially boom your danger of fractures.

Many alkaline-weight-reduction plan proponents believe that to preserve a consistent blood pH, your frame takes alkaline minerals, such as calcium out of your bones, to buffer the acids from the acid-forming ingredients you consume.

In step with this concept, acid-forming diets, which includes the standard Western food plan, will cause a loss in bone mineral density. This concept is known as the "acid-ash hypothesis of osteoporosis."

But, this theory ignores the characteristic of your kidneys, which can be fundamental to eliminating acids and regulating body pH.

The kidneys produce bicarbonate ions that neutralize acids to your blood, allowing your body to closely manipulate blood pH.

Your respiratory device is also worried in controlling blood pH. While bicarbonate ions from your kidneys bind to acids for your blood, they shape carbon dioxide, which you breathe out, and water, which you pee out.

The acid-ash speculation additionally ignores one of the

major drivers of osteoporosis — a loss within the protein collagen from bone.

Ironically, this loss of collagen is strongly linked to low ranges of acids — orthosilicic acid and ascorbic acid, or diet C — on your food plan.

Remember that clinical proof linking nutritional acid to bone density or fracture danger is blended. At the same time as many observational studies have located no affiliation, others have detected a sizable link.

Scientific trials, which tend to be extra correct, have concluded that acid-forming diets don't have any effect on calcium ranges for your body.

If something, these diets enhance bone fitness by way of increasing calcium retention and activating the IGF-1 hormone, which stimulates the restore of muscle and bone.

As such, a excessive-protein, acid-forming food regimen is probable

connected to better bone health —
now not worse.

Summary

Although proof is mixed, most
studies does now not help the
principle that acid-forming diets
harm your bones. Protein, an
acidic nutrient, even seems to be
useful.

Acidity and cancer

Many human beings argue that
cancer handiest grows in an acidic
surroundings and may be treated
oreven cured with an alkaline
eating regimen.

However, comprehensive opinions on the connection among eating regimen-precipitated acidosis — or accelerated blood acidity due to food regimen — and cancer concluded that there's no direct hyperlink.

First, meals doesn't substantially affect blood pH.

Second, even in case you expect that meals may want to dramatically regulate the pH cost of blood or different tissues, cancer cells are not constrained to acidic environments.

In fact, cancer grows in ordinary body tissue, which has a slightly alkaline pH of seven. Four. Many experiments have correctly grown cancer cells in an alkaline environment.

And whilst tumors grow quicker in acidic environments, tumors create this acidity themselves. It isn't the acidic environment that creates most cancers cells, but cancer cells that create the acidic environment.

Precis

There's no link among an acid-forming food plan and cancer. Cancer cells also grow in alkaline environments.

Akaline diets and acidity
Analyzing the acid-alkaline idea from each an evolutionary and clinical attitude exhibits discrepancies.

One examine expected that 87% of pre-agricultural human beings ate alkaline diets and shaped the imperative argument at the back of the present day alkaline eating regimen.

Greater latest studies approximates that half of pre-agricultural human beings ate net alkaline-forming diets, at the same time as the alternative 1/2 ate internet acid-forming diets.

Remember the fact that our faraway ancestors lived in massively extraordinary climates with get admission to to numerous ingredients. In fact, acid-forming diets had been more commonplace as human beings moved in addition north of the equator, far from the tropics.

Although around 1/2 of hunter-gatherers were ingesting a internet acid-forming weight-reduction plan, cutting-edge diseases are believed to had been lots much less common.

Summary

Present day research advocate that about 1/2 of Akaline diets have been acid-forming, specially among folks that lived some distance from the equator.

The bottom line

The alkaline weight loss plan is pretty healthy, encouraging a excessive intake of fruits, vegetables, and healthful plant foods whilst restricting processed junk foods.

However, the perception that the weight-reduction plan boosts fitness because of its alkalizing results is suspect. These claims haven't been verified via any dependable human studies.

A few research propose nice effects in a completely small subset of the populace. Specially, a low-protein alkalizing weight loss plan might also benefit people with persistent kidney disorder.

In widespread, the alkaline weight loss program is healthful because it's based totally on whole and unprocessed meals. No reliable evidence shows it has anything to do with pH ranges.

CHAPTER 2
Hints for restricting Acidic foods

Defining acidity

The pH value tells you if some thing is an acid, a base, or impartial.

A pH of zero indicates a high degree of acidity.

A pH of 7 is impartial.

A pH of 14 is the most basic, or alkaline.

As an example, battery acid is extremely acidic at 0, at the same time as liquid drain cleanser is very alkaline at 14. Natural distilled water is within the middle at 7. It's neither acidic nor alkaline.

Much like extraordinary materials, specific elements of the human body have special pH stages. Your ideal blood pH is among 7.35 and seven.Forty five, that's slightly alkaline. The stomach is usually at a pH of 3.5, which enables food ruin down well.

High-acid food and drink

In case you suspect you have got issues with acidity, you may make adjustments to your food regimen to assist enhance signs and symptoms. Meals which are taken into consideration acidic should have a pH degree of 4.6 or decrease.

Meals that tend to cause greater acidity in the frame and that you may want to restrict or avoid consist of:

Grains

Sugar

Certain dairy products

Fish

Processed ingredients

Sparkling meats and processed meats, inclusive of corned pork and turkey

Sodas and other sweetened liquids

Excessive-protein foods and dietary supplements

Studies supporting the connection between foods like animal protein and dairy and persistent disease due to a alternate in the frame's pH is restricted. New research may also shed extra mild in this connection, or disclose other reasons why reducing animal products is beneficial for fitness.

Right here's a list of culmination and their pH from Clemson college. They're indexed from most acidic to least:

Lemon juice (pH: 2.00–2.60)

Limes (pH: 2.00–2.80)

Blue plums (pH: 2.80–3.40)

Grapes (pH: 2.Ninety–3.82)

Pomegranates (pH: 2.93–3.20)

Grapefruits (pH: 3.00–three.75)

Blueberries (pH: 3.12–three.33)

Pineapples (pH: three.20–4.00)

Apples (pH: three.30–4.00)

Peaches (pH: three.30–4.05)

Oranges (pH: 3.69–4.34)

Tomatoes (pH: four.30–four.90)

Normally, citrus fruits have a low pH, which means they are acidic. Citrus and other acidic foods can also make a contribution to symptoms in people with top gastrointestinal troubles like an ulcer or reflux.

It's crucial to keep in mind that fruit juices are acidic, too. Due to this, you have to use a straw while consuming fruit juices. This keeps the fruit juice from coming in direct contact along with your teeth.

If fruit doesn't aggravate upper digestive symptoms, they may be a wholesome meals to devour daily and were proven to lessen continual disorder chance. Despite their initial acidity, maximum end result are alkalizing.

Vegetables, particularly fresh veggies, are usually no longer taken into consideration acidic. Right here's a listing of vegetables and their pH ranges:

Sauerkraut (pH: 3.30–3.60)

Cabbage (pH: five.20–6.Eighty)

Beets (pH: five.30–6.60)

Corn (pH: five.90–7.50)

Mushrooms (pH: 6.00–6.70)

Broccoli (pH: 6.30-6.85)

Collard vegetables (pH: 6.50–7.50)

You can pick out to keep away from high-phosphorus liquids such as beer or hot chocolate crafted from packets of cocoa mix. Mineral sodas or glowing water may be an excellent replacement. In case you do desire to drink alcohol, go with lower phosphorus red or white wine.

In terms of the blessings of a greater alkaline food regimen, studies published in the journal of Environmental and Public HealthTrusted supply says that no conclusive evidence shows it improves bone fitness. However, it is able to assist limit muscle loss, fortify reminiscence and alertness, and help you stay longer.

Some alkalizing (or impartial) foods and liquids you could include into your eating regimen encompass:

Soy, along with miso, soy beans, tofu, and tempeh

Unsweetened yogurt and milk

Maximum clean veggies, which includes potatoes

Maximum fruits

Herbs and spices, with the exception of salt, mustard, and nutmeg

Some whole grains, inclusive of millet, quinoa, and amaranth

Herbal teas

Fat like olive oil, avocados, nuts, and seeds

Effects of consuming too many acid-producing ingredients

A food regimen that includes too many acid-producing foods, which include protein or sugar, can motive acidity for your urine in addition to different negative fitness consequences. This may motive a kind of kidney stone referred to as uric acid stones to form.

It's been speculated that too much acidity also can cause bone and muscle deterioration. That is because bones contain calcium, which your frame uses to restore your blood's pH balance whilst it turns into too acidic.

Some proof suggests that phosphoric acid, commonly discovered in darker sodas, is connected to decrease bone density, particularly when it replaces milk, a calcium- and protein-rich beverage. Too much acidity can also boom your danger for most cancers, liver issues, and coronary heart disease.

Some foods and drinks produce less acid than sodas or protein, but they nonetheless don't offer the foremost alkalizing impact of most fruits and veggies. Experts don't always agree on the exact meals lists.

Aim to limit these ingredients considering that they will be affecting your acid-base stability or affecting your fitness in negative ways:

Corn oil

Sweeteners, together with sugar, molasses, maple syrup, processed honey, and aspartame

Salt

Condiments, which include mayonnaise, soy sauce, and vinegar

Hard and processed cheeses

Grains, such as corn, rice, and wheat

In case you're involved about acid wearing down bone, you may take small amounts of sodium bicarbonate. College of California, San Diego, researchers advise doses which might be less than 5 grams.

You shouldn't take sodium bicarbonate for the duration of mealtimes due to the fact it could interfere along with your digestion. Getting enough nutritional calcium, nutrition D, phosphorus, and magnesium can also be useful for offsetting the terrible outcomes of acid for your bone.

Prevention

Because waste merchandise have a tendency to be acidic, researchers at the college of California in San Diego suggest ingesting extra assets of alkaline-generating meals, along with end result and vegetables, at a 3-to-1 ratio. The pH of a food before you consume it's miles much less vital than what it turns into once it's inner your body.

At the same time as uncommon, it's feasible for the urine's pH to be too alkaline. But, in the u.S., too much acid has a tendency to be a extra not unusual trouble. This is because of the high charges at which human beings devour animal protein, sugar, and grains. Higher fees of prescription drug use also contribute to the trouble.

Takeaway

The alkaline food regimen is a healthful alternative that may fit due extra to the emphasis on consuming flora and restricting processed foods than to converting the frame's pH.

Eating extra fruits and vegetables, along side curtailing your refined carbohydrate, sugar, and dairy intake, might also or might not help stability pH tiers within your body.

Both way, a plant-heavy diet with reduced refined sugar intake has many fitness benefits and can reduce day by day troubles and decrease the opportunity of certain lengthy-term health dangers.